22 TIPS TO LOSE WEIGHT:

SMALL CHANGES WITH BIG RESULTS

@Weightloss_Solution6

Table of Contents

Introduction

Most of us are creatures of habit. We buy the same foods from the same grocery store, prepare the same recipes over and over, and live within our familiar routines. But if you're serious about eating healthier and losing weight, you need to shake it up, change those bad eating habits, and start thinking differently about your diet and lifestyle.

The problem is that we get so comfortable in our ways that it's hard to give up those old habits.

Another expert notes that you're much more likely to be successful at changing your habits if you take things one step at a time. "Try to gradually incorporate new habits over time, and before you know it, you will be eating more healthfully and losing weight," says Keri Gans, MS, RD, American Dietetic Association spokesperson and a nutritionist in private practice in New York.

Making a few small changes to your morning habits can be an easy and effective way to increase weight loss.

Practicing healthy behaviors in the morning can also get your day started on the right foot and set you up for success.

For best results, make sure you combine these morning habits with a well-rounded diet and a healthy lifestyle.

Chapter 1:
Change your habits and your goals

Prioritization. It is crucial to identify your key motivations and list them according to priorities.

Become More Mindful. One of the first steps toward conquering lousy eating habits is paying more attention to what you're eating and drinking. "Read food labels, become familiar with lists of ingredients, and start to take notice of everything you put into your mouth," says Gans. Once you become more aware of what you're eating, you'll start to realize how you need to improve your diet. Some people benefit from keeping food diaries.

Healthy people in our culture are aware of what they're putting in their bodies. Unhealthy people willingly choose to live in blissful ignorance. In the information age that we live in, we must educate ourselves on what we're eating.

Nutrition labels aren't perfect, but they're useful. They make you aware of additives and other strange ingredients, and they also help you to understand how many calories you're about to consume. It is essential to note.

One of the reasons you may be struggling with excess weight around your mid-section is because you're consuming too many calories. The average healthy diet allows for the consumption of approximately 2,000 calories/day, depending on your activity level. If you're eating, drinking, and snacking on the wrong foods all day long, you're very likely eating well over 2,000 calories. Some days you may be easily doubling that amount.

If your caloric intake is too high, it would be a wise and beneficial habit to take a closer look at food labels, not only for the sake of avoiding unhealthy additives and ingredients but also for the sake of understanding your daily level of calorie consumption

Make a daily Plan; Be Specific. How are you going to start eating more fruit, having breakfast every day, or getting to the gym more often? Spell out your options. For example, Plan to take a piece of fruit to work every day for snacks, stock up on cereal and fruit for quick breakfasts, and go to the gym on the way to work three times a week. "To say 'I am going to work out more,' won't help you," says Gans. "What will help is thinking about when and how you can fit it into your lifestyle."

Tackle a New Mini-Goal Each Week. These mini-steps will eventually add up to significant change. One of the bad habits we often engage in is the tendency to establish unreasonable goals for ourselves in our weight loss journey. We start the week by saying, "OK, this week; I am going to lose 7 lbs." Then at the end of the week, we step on the scale and get disappointed because we only lost 3 lbs.

It's important to set reasonable goals. We all have the long-term plan in mind of having the perfect physique, but in the meantime, let's do ourselves the favor of setting some short-term goals that are achievable and worth celebrating.

Get in the habit of setting reasonable goals and then celebrating when you reach them. Be patient with yourself, and show yourself an ample amount of grace. It is a marathon, not a sprint.

Be Realistic. Don't expect too much from yourself too soon. It takes about a month for any new action to become a habit. Slow and steady wins the race -- along with a dose of vigilance.

Chapter 2:
Hold Yourself Accountable

Hold yourself accountable: willpower alone is not always enough to ensure long-term success. That's where accountability is essential. It helps you stay on the right path for weight loss success and allows you to make adjustments along the way.

One way to stay accountable is to weigh yourself more frequently. Research has shown that people who weigh themselves more regularly are more likely to lose weight and keep it off, compared with people who don't weight themselves as often (21Trusted Source). Weigh yourself before you start the plan so that you can see your daily, weekly, and monthly progress until you reach your goal. Please write down your weight, your daily exercise, and how many minutes you did it, and the food that you ate. It will help you keep track of your progress from day one. Seeing your progress will help you be motivated to go on to see how far you have gone or how far you still need to go. Include your before and after photos so you could see the difference.

Another way to stay accountable is to keep a food journal. It allows you to keep track of your food intake, which can help you lose weight and keep it off longer (22Trusted Source, 23Trusted Source).

Lastly, you could try partnering with a friend who has similar weight loss goals or joining an in-person or online weight loss community. Doing so can not only help you with your plan but also make things fun to help keep you motivated (24Trusted Source). Once you have decided to commit to meditation to weight loss, don't shy away from sharing your plan with your support system and family. It is to ensure that the people you share with also reinforce the commitment and form part of the support system. That way, they will feel part of the program and give support whenever there is a need. You can also use apps for reminders and timings; this way, you have a backup plan whenever you forget. You can also use motivational bands whenever you achieve a milestone set. Being accountable makes you enjoy your successes, acknowledge your failure, and appreciate your support system. People thrive when they feel responsible for something, especially on something beneficial to their well-being.

Chapter 3:
Practice Stress Management

"Focus on dealing with stress through exercise, relaxation, meditation, or whatever works for you, so you don't fall back into those bad habits during periods of stress or use food to help you cope with the situation," advises Foreyt.

Stress eating affects millions of people each year, and although not many will admit it can cause food addiction and unhealthy eating choices. As one eats, they believe eating relieve them of stress and often blame other people for their problems. They do not take responsibility for their actions. They do not see the need to eat healthy because their mind is preoccupied with so many things.

Having a stress management technique should be part of one's daily routine. You need to develop a healthy stress-relieving mechanism that can help you live a stress-free life. Understand that meditation is a stress reliever in its own right as it helps calm the mind and soothes the body. It can be used to manage stress and its benefits fully utilized to live a more productive life. Be able to handle stress efficiently. Stress is not healthy for the mind. If not controlled, it can cause emotional problems and makes one irrational, moody, or violent. Be your boss when managing your stress.

It happens when people start overeating or under food when they are overwhelmed with mixed emotions rather than eating in response to their inner cues. Strong emotions we experience can sometimes prevent us from listening to our physical feelings and thus preventing us from feeling hungry or full. This habit is very addictive, and if not controlled, can lead to obesity, rapid weight gain, overeating, guilt, and shame. Stress-related eating disorder, if not handled, can make one vulnerable and not comfortable with their body. It is where meditation plays a significant role because one will be able to manage their stress situation and, therefore, not use food as a coping mechanism. Stress eating affects millions of people each year, and although not many will admit it can cause food addiction and unhealthy eating choices. As one eats, they believe eating relieve them of stress and often blame other people for their problems. They do not take responsibility for their actions.

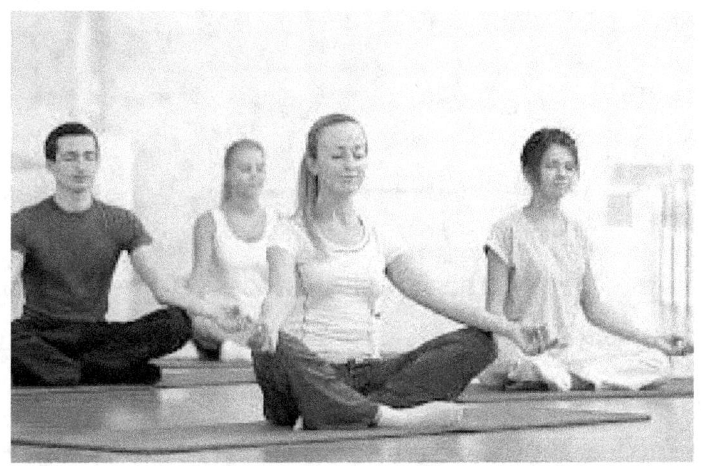

Chapter 4:
Eat a High-Protein Breakfast

The reason breakfast is considered the most important meal of the day. Eating a high-protein breakfast may help cut cravings and aid in weight loss, high-protein breakfast may aid weight loss by reducing cravings, appetite and ghrelin secretion

A healthy breakfast should be balanced and deliver a mix of protein, complex carbohydrates, fiber, and healthy fat to keep you full and fueled up for your day.

Preferred: Healthy Breakfast Recipes including

- Raspberries
- Oatmeal
- Yogurt
- Peanut Butter
- Eggs

Most people agree that breakfast is a pretty substantial meal. Of all the meals in the day, it's the meal when you can let yourself indulge a little. It can provide a nice energy boost, increase morning productivity, and help you resist the urge to over-indulge at lunchtime.

All that being said, it may be that you're in the habit of eating the wrong things for breakfast. If your breakfast typically consists of things like cereals (even some of the so-called "healthy" ones), donuts, toast, muffins, jelly, biscuits, and other starchy or sugary foods, you're actually in the habit of increasing your belly fat, not reducing it.

Instead of indulging in these sugary, carby, and starchy foods, consider eating a breakfast that incorporates more proteins, nuts, fruits, and vegetables. It is a pattern of eating that we would do well to utilize throughout the day. Omelets, sliced fruit, and smoothies are great options to get the day started. Even breakfast meats like bacon, sausage, and ham can help contribute to the loss of belly fat when enjoyed in moderation.

The reason we struggle to make eating a "smart" breakfast a daily habit is because it takes more planning than eating cereals, toasts, muffins, and donuts. But filling up on proteins, nuts, fruits, and veggies keeps us feeling full longer and can help us control our appetite well into the day.

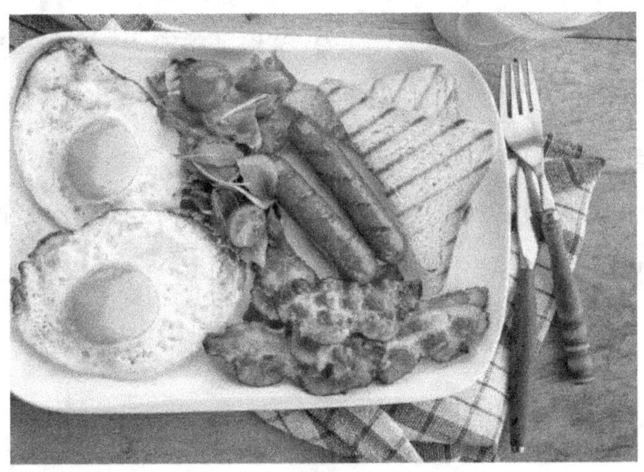

Chapter 5:
Prepare your food in advance

Making an effort to plan and pack your meals ahead of time can be a simple way to make better food choices and increase weight loss.

Try setting aside a few hours one night a week to plan and prepare your meals so that in the morning, you can just grab your lunch and go.

Preparing your lunch the day before or in the morning may seem like a tedious task, but it can save you a lot of money in the long run, and it will also help you to understand what goes into your body. Making your lunch also gives you perfect control of your portions and the ingredients of whatever you are eating.

If you don't carry lunch to work, chances are you are going to go out and buy food. The cheapest alternative is usually something from the local fast-food restaurant. Buying a burger, fries, and soda combo for lunch is a bit overkill and unhealthy. Another problem with not carrying lunch at work can be an inconvenience. What happens on the day you are too busy to go out for lunch? You will probably end up skipping lunch. The problem with skipping lunch is that you could end up overeating or overcompensating later on in the day.

Chapter 6:
Start Tracking Your Intake

Keeping a food diary to track what you eat can be an effective way to help boost weight loss and hold yourself accountable.

Keep more fruits, low-fat dairy products (low-fat milk and low-fat yogurt), vegetables, and wholegrain foods at home and at work. ...

Try to eat a family meal every day at the kitchen or dining table.

Buy a healthy-recipe book, and cook for yourself.

Chew gum when you cook so you will not be tempted to snack on the ingredients.

Eat your meals with others when you can. Relax and enjoy your meals, and do not eat too fast. Try to make healthy eating a pleasure, not a chore.

This habit of tracking your progress, I feel, is one of the easiest, yet most powerful tips you can add to your weight loss journey. I say this because if you have been applying all the advice we discussed up to this point, you already can see and feel that you're losing weight. At this time, all you have to do now is track down how much weight you have lost or what you have done to help your weight loss. Tracking can be done in a variety of ways. For instance, you can download a weight-loss mobile app and track the foods you have eaten during the day.

It is a helpful tool because these types of apps provide you access to see how many calories you have consumed, what foods you are consuming, and some even offer options to add to your weight loss routine. Another way to track your progress is by journaling or documenting your progress daily. This process is when you physically write down your progress in a journal or document your progression in other matters, such as using your phone to track. Tracking your progress this way helps you see different things you have been doing throughout the day on your weight loss journey. Some examples of this could be that today you were able to do a 30 min walk, you were able to drink more water, or better yet, you were able to lose 5lb in a month!

Tracking your progress this way and using mobile apps are both effective ways to keep up on how you are doing amid your journey. The reason that tracking your progress is so important is that you have to see yourself doing good to keep doing good. Also, research has shown people who do this are more likely to stay on a weight loss regimen. Just picture it, you have been applying weight-loss tactics for a month, you can see that you're doing good because you have been tracking your success; how would you feel? I would say pretty incredible and this would motivate you to go further in your weight loss journey to lose my weight!

To conclude, tracking your progress is not hard to do and can promote a lot towards your weight loss goals. Do not overthink this process; track down everything you do during your weight loss journey and look back at what you have done to improve. In essence, tracking your progress is a reinforcement tactic to reinforce all the positive actions you have done, which will boost your mindset during your weight loss journey.

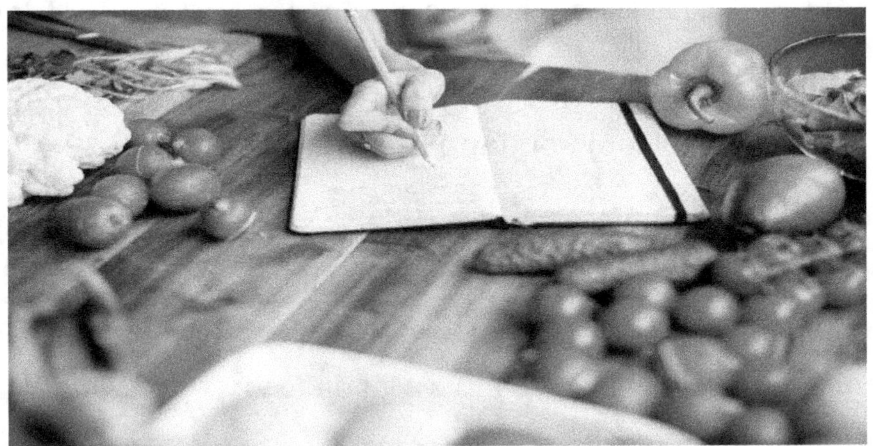

Chapter 7:
Eat often and at an optimal time

You should eat every 2-3 hours 5-7 times per day (small meals)

Should eat within one hour of waking up, also preferred to eat thirty minutes before working out

Do not skip or delay meals, and be sure to schedule your snacks. If you ignore your feelings of hunger, you may end up overeating or choosing an unhealthy snack. If you often feel hungry, it can cause you to focus a lot on food.

It is yet another trick to convince your body that food is plentiful. If your body thinks food is plentiful, then it has no reason to store it! Eating more regularly will maintain a stable level of blood sugar and a more consistent supply of energy. Be careful not to eat more during the day as a result of this. Don't eat extra snacks; just spread out the food you would typically eat. If you have fruit and yogurt with lunch, then have the fruit mid-morning and the yogurt mid-afternoon.

Regular eating will help to keep your metabolism in an excellent zone, steadily burning up your fat reserves. Don't be tempted to skip breakfast or any other meal. I know how easy it is to become busy or so involved in an activity that it becomes difficult to have that snack or meal at just the right time. That's why it's essential to plan ahead and always make sure you have a snack with you.

If your friends are meeting for coffee and cake, or there is a morning tea at work, pack your snack and have it with the rest of the group or, if you feel uncomfortable doing that, eat it in private. Don't be shy about refusing a slice of that lovely cake your friend has made: your friends or associates will accept that you're trying to lose weight. You can still enjoy a cup of coffee. If you have an activity in the evening, carry your snack along in a little snack bag. Your friends will envy your self-control and be happy to help in any way they can.

Chapter 8:
Thermogenic intake, be a pain-Free Naturally

Support the desired weight loss through temperature workings by increasing body temperature and metabolism, which increase energy levels; thus, more calories are utilized.

Thermogenesis is an advanced scientific concept, but simply means how increasing the consumption of some substances can help speed metabolism, burn fat, and ultimately lead to significant weight loss. Thermogenics are a class of supplements that access a variety of methods to raise a person's metabolism. By presenting a person's metabolism, weight loss, if done correctly, is the result.

The amount of activity that you do every day and your choice of food intake also play vital roles in how your body uses its sources in burning fat. You will need to convert the food you intake into energy to aid the process. This process of converting food into energy is called metabolism.

Every person has a specific metabolic rate, which is why one individual may lose weight faster than the others. By improving and controlling your metabolism, you are also improving your body's fat-burning capabilities

Thermogenesis influences the body's metabolic rate and leads to an increase in fat and calories burned. When stimulated, thermogenic can concurrently increase a person's energy levels and help speed fat oxidation. Thermogenics are enhanced by the ingestion of various substances, including bitter orange, ephedra, capsicum, ginger, and pyruvate. Caffeine and EGCG found in green tea extract also increase Thermogenesis.

Thermogenic supplements are taken as a daily dietary supplement or before weight training or cardiovascular activity and provide a long-lasting burst of energy to help optimize performance and increase the results of dieting.

The addition of green tea extract, bitter orange, and other ingredients are excellent compounds that can enhance Thermogenesis. Although bodybuilders, athletes, and weightlifters have historically been the primary consumers of thermogenic products, these additives are now entering the mainstream dieting industry at a feverish pace.

Weight loss and burning fat are now realistic results by regularly ingesting nutritional products that enhance Thermogenesis.

Chapter 9:
Take your Multivitamins and lake of nutrition

Nearly 81% of US health professionals take multivitamins regularly.But while multivitamins generally help individuals supplement their deficiencies, they also have their downsides as well.

The largest problem with multivitamins is that they are not always of high quality. Typically the average amount of vitamin D in a vitamin pill is inadequate, the magnesium is of low quality, and of course, there is no omega 3 in multivitamins. Cheap vitamin pills are less expensive because of the low standards presented in the bottle.

Nevertheless, supplementing vitamin and mineral intake with quality multivitamins is an excellent strategy to start with for those that believe they have a deficiency. Because they are commonly found in your nearest drugstore, multivitamins enable you to experience beneficial results rapidly. But just as it goes with physical exercise, the easiest solution leads to a plateau, and you will then need to replenish the three significant nutrient deficiencies.

So who should take micronutrient supplements? Well, it is recommended that every adult over the age of 40 take regular supplements without a doubt. However, even if you are younger, you can undoubtedly benefit from supplementation.

Chapter 10:
Take your Omega3, zinc, magnesium, vitamin D

Some studies have concluded that specific vitamins and minerals might be excellent aids in weight loss efforts through various means. Take, for example, zinc, which aids in the production of the hormone leptin, which, in turn, will make you feel full and, hence, you would end up eating less. Other studies have shown that women post-menopause who took calcium and vitamin D managed to control their weight better than others who did not take the vitamin. Also, check out chromium, which is a mineral with a strong reputation as a weight loss aid as well as a muscle mass builder.

Omega3 – a compound most abundant in fish oil - is immensely popular due to its many benefits. It reduces inflammation, helps with depression, regulates blood pressure, and reduces blood cholesterol. Studies also have shown that the Omega3 fatty acids are highly beneficial for preventing, arresting, and even reversing Alzheimer's and dementia in senior people.

As a weight loss aid supplement, Omega3 fatty acids have been found to help regulate blood sugar and insulin levels, accelerate the burning of fat and suppress hunger by preventing the production of certain enzymes whose roles are to store fat in the body.

Magnesium is a mineral that has traditionally been a little underrated, but researchers now realize just how essential it is. For example, they've recently learned that all that calcium you've been taking to help build strong bones can't be adequately metabolized unless you're getting enough magnesium to go with it.

When it comes to boosting your metabolism and losing weight, magnesium is also essential. It's responsible for regulating blood sugar, heartbeat, and muscle contractions. In other words, every time you flex a muscle or lift a pen, that's magnesium at work.

The regulation of blood sugar is the main advantage here. By keeping your blood sugar steady, magnesium helps reduce between-meal cravings and allows your body to use the fuel from a meal more efficiently, meaning less of it ends up getting stored as fat.

Some of the healthiest foods that contain magnesium are listed below:

- Any assortment of nuts
- Any assortment of seeds
- Beans and chickpeas
- Kale and spinach

One of the most impressive things about vitamin D is that it slows the formation of new fat cells, meaning you avoid putting those extra pounds on in the first place. In addition to slowing the formation of fat, vitamin D also increases the number of calories you're burning, even at rest. So, altogether, it's boosting your fat burning goals on both sides of the equation.

The absolute best way to get vitamin D is to just go outside in the sunlight. It's a zero-calorie option and comes with plenty of other great benefits. Given enough sunlight, you can absorb and create enough Vitamin D for your body. If that isn't enough reason to get outside, that sunlight will also boost your metabolism on its own. Studies have shown that a few minutes of daylight can speed up your calorie burn significantly and that the effects will last for as long as an hour after you've gone back inside.

How much sunlight you need to make enough vitamin D depends but is usually somewhere between 10-30 minutes. Make sure you use plenty of sunscreens, though. Sunscreen will protect your skin from damage while still allowing your body to manufacture vitamin D and speed up its metabolism.

If you're concerned, you aren't able to get your 10-30 minutes of sunlight each day; you can find some foods that have been fortified with vitamin D to make up for this lack.

Some of the healthiest sources of vitamin D fortified foods include:

- Cod Liver Oil
- Sardines
- Tuna
- Salmon
- Eggs
- Milk
- Yogurt

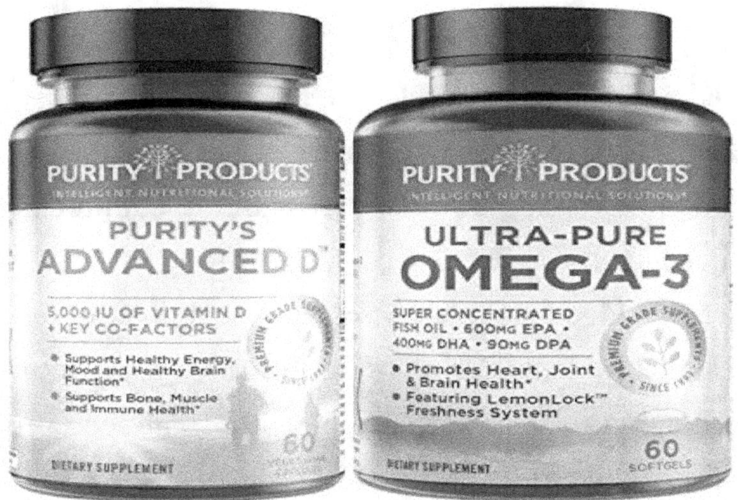

Chapter 11:
Drink to fitness

Water is one of the main elements required to sustain life all over the world. Therefore naturally, water intake is highly essential for a healthy body. Start drinking that water! And make sure you keep track of your daily water intake. At least 8-10 glasses of water are recommended for the average human, and there should be no compromise on that level.

Keeping your body hydrated helps the metabolism remain regulated and also helps to cleanse the body on the inside. Due to an increase in exercise while performing any diet, the loss of water due to sweating also increases, and to counter that loss, water needs to be replenished within the body. Furthermore, one of the added benefits of water is that it is excellent for curing skin problems. Drinking more water prevents the skin from becoming too dry and also helps to treat acne problems. Especially to the girls, water is your best friend, so don't leave it out of your diets. Drink up, everyone, no diet is complete without maintaining an adequate water intake!

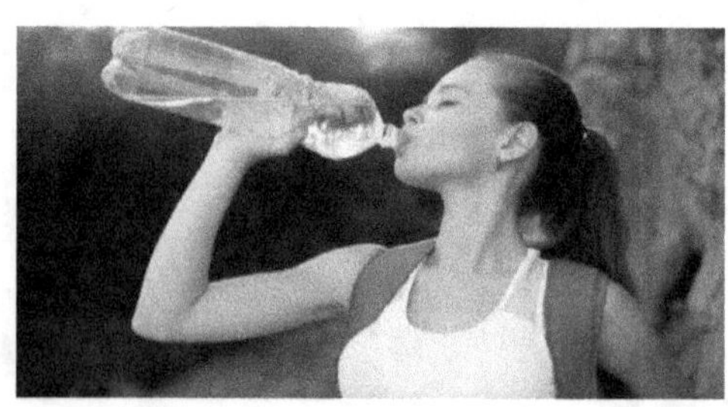

Chapter 12:
Weigh Yourself

Stepping on the scale and weighing yourself each morning (one time a day) can be an effective method to increase motivation and improve self-control.

Weighing yourself, every morning can also help foster healthy habits and behaviors that may promote weight loss.

Additionally, remember that your weight may fluctuate daily and can be influenced by a variety of factors. Focus on the big picture and look for overall weight loss trends, rather than getting fixated on small day-to-day changes.

It is easier to remember to weigh yourself daily - you get into the habit of weighing yourself.

The key is to weigh yourself at the same time EVERY MORNING – that is the only right way to keep track of how you are progressing. I find it's easiest to weigh myself as soon as I get out of bed.

That way, you have no excuses about having eaten something "heavy" or having had too many cups of tea. Your weight will fluctuate throughout the day and may even fluctuate from day to day.

If you want an accurate of your progress, you must weigh yourself at the same time every day, when your body is in a similar state to what it was before.

The other reason why weighing yourself daily is essential is that it is quite motivating. While we know intellectually that the movement on the scale is not necessarily indicative of weight loss, you do start to see patterns after tracking for at least a week.

You'll know straight away if something has gone seriously wrong with the plan, instead of only finding out three or four days later and doing even more damage.

You'll be more inclined to "behave" if you've weighed yourself in the morning. Either the results will be motivating because you pick up losses straight away or you get scared straight because you've been bad.

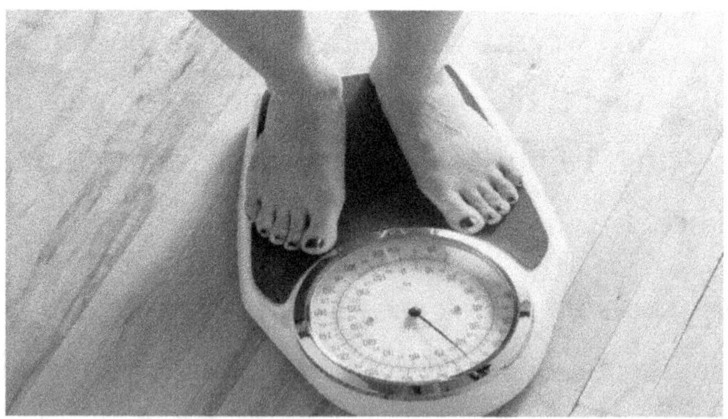

Chapter13:
Some Exercises

Getting in some physical activity first thing in the morning can help boost weight loss.

Exercising in the morning may also help keep blood sugar levels steady throughout the day. Low blood sugar can result in many negative symptoms, including excessive hunger.

Early Morning Freshness Advantage

Being able to have a proper schedule where one can condition him or herself to wake up early in the morning is very important to maintain a healthy lifestyle. Mornings are known to radiate freshness and are a great way to start any weight loss regime. The body is well-rested, which is exceptionally crucial to able to start the day with energy and vigor. Waking up early in the morning helps the body to set a fixed, regular, and efficient routine for its self. It allows the body to get rid of that feeling of constant fatigue and laziness that usually happens due to a lack of a properly functioning daily routine. Lastly, it helps to regulate the metabolism and prevents it from becoming lax and slowing down.

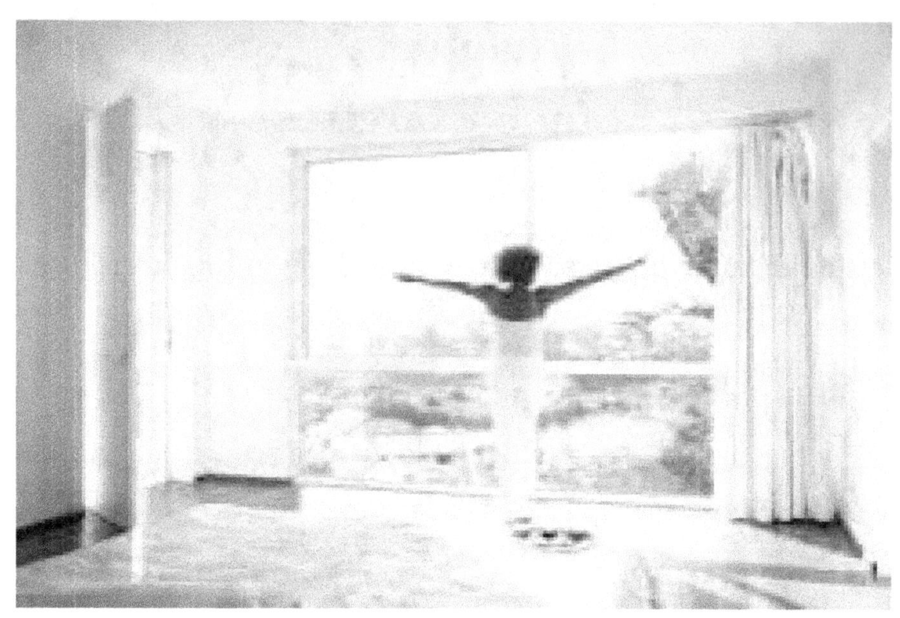

First Crucial Body Stretch

People often tend to undermine the significance of body stretches, forgetting the fact for the body to be able to perform any activity efficiently; it needs to have all its muscles in good condition. So immediately after waking up, doing your morning stretches is a must! Work your way downwards, simple neck rotary movements, and side to side movements followed by the arm stretches along with shoulder rolling. Then twist your upper body that is waist upwards sideways on each side at least fifteen to twenty times. Lastly, come to the leg stretches, move each leg separately sideways, back and forth along with moving the feet in a rotator motion at the ankle joint. A whole well-performed body stretch will help lose all that laziness and prepare the body for any exercise to come!

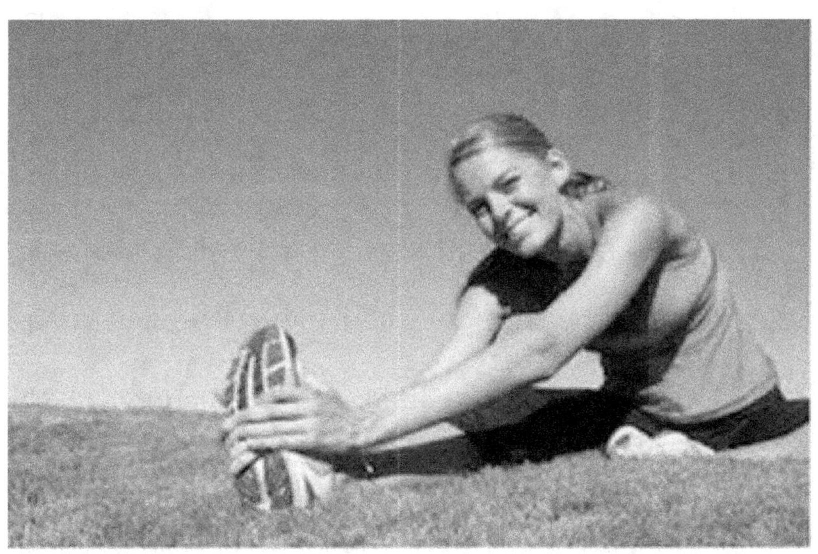

Early Morning Exercise Benefits

No weight loss program is complete without exercise for obvious reasons, of course. Training is the best most effective way to not only shed those extra pounds but also to keep the body healthy. It allows the body to maintain itself and regulates the metabolism so that it keeps working appropriately. Exercise strengthens muscles also and keeps the body active and energetic. Controlling the amount of weight to be lost, an exercise schedule should be drawn up comprising of cycling 15-20 minutes daily, 15-20 minutes of walking/treadmill daily, jump roping, or even simple moves like jumping jacks are good enough. Morning exercise rejuvenates and makes one more active.

Chapter 14:
Sleep Well

Going to bed a bit earlier or setting your alarm clock later to squeeze in some extra sleep may help increase weight loss.

Lack of sleep has also been linked to an increase in calorie intake.

The body has a natural rhythm that we would do well to pay attention to. We have been designed to consume a certain amount of calories during the day and then rest at night. If we aren't getting the kind of sleep we need, we tend to throw off this rhythm and put ourselves in a position where our bodies are going to function in more of a deprivation mode.

Sleep is an essential part of health that shouldn't be ignored. When we develop the habit of getting ample sleep (6.5 - 8 hours/night), we have more energy for the tasks of the day. Likewise, our stress levels are lessened, and our emotional resistance to over-eating is strengthened.

When we get enough sleep, our motivation level tends to remain higher as well. But our culture doesn't value sleep as it ought to. We love "burning the midnight oil" instead of enjoying adequate rest, and we pride ourselves on telling others that we don't require as much sleep as they do.

But if you ask a majority of those who have consistently maintained a healthy weight for long periods of time, you will notice a pattern in their answers. Most people who are successful with their weight loss and maintenance goals are also getting enough sleep each evening. This is an important habit that we cannot overlook.

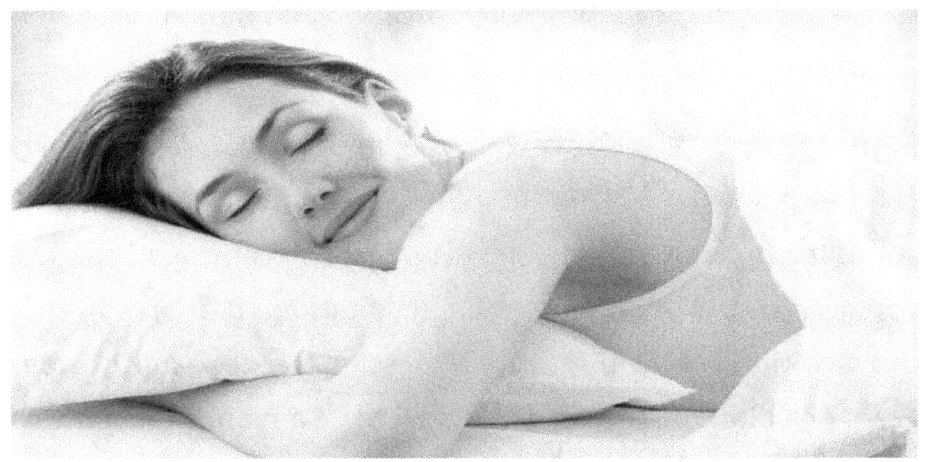

Chapter 15:
Meditation and Avoid stress

The first technique is good old mindfulness meditation, which now has scientific evidence showing the benefits of reducing stress as well as altering the brain, genes, and behavior. (Kaliman)

Start the day peacefully with meditation, and it will carry through your day. In recent times, meditation has become a widespread habit. These days there are many applications, courses, and classes that teach meditation. It is a powerful practice that can help reduce depression, anxiety, and various mental health issues. You don't need to be a monk or a spiritual person to gain the benefits of meditation. It works the same for all of us, and it doesn't matter who you are or what you do.

Regular meditation enhances your brain and helps you to deal with stress much more effectively. Not only that, but it provides numerous mental health benefits from concentration to calmness and much more. Scientists have also observed that meditation causes your brain to release endorphins. These are the chemicals that make us feel good.

Morning is the best time for meditation because your mind is alert and less prone to distractions. There is less stress at this time of day, especially if you have followed the morning routine and have not used your phone yet. If you need more time for meditation, then wake up a little bit earlier. If your too busy, then that means you need it! You will be grateful for all the benefits it provides.

To begin, sit in a comfortable place that is quiet and free from distractions. The best position is to sit cross-legged. But if that's uncomfortable for you, then you can lie down or sit in a chair. Wear some comfortable clothes and have the right temperature setting. You don't want to be getting up or moving around during your meditation sessions. Some people find value from further blocking out noise and light using eye masks and noise-canceling headphones. These will allow you to go into a deep meditative state. Try them if you like.

Set a timer on your phone and turn the data off. If your a beginner, start with five minutes and then, after some weeks or months of practice, increase the time. The best results come from fifteen to thirty-minute sessions. Eyes can be open or closed as you wish. Then you simply breathe in and out. Focus on your breath going in and out of your body. Relax and let your breath flow. Allow your breathing to find its rhythm. Just be.

Stay like this until your alarm goes off. If thoughts enter into your mind, just watch them pass by. If you catch yourself engaging in thoughts, then become aware, let them go, and come back again to your breathing. If a sound or anything else distracts you, let it go and again come back to your breathing.

There are many more styles of mediation. Some involve focusing on breathing while others repeat words/mantras, and then some even combine meditation with yoga. It's a vast subject and has only been covered briefly here. If you are interested to learn more, then I suggest checking out some YouTube videos or study a course.

Breathing Exercises

Breathing exercises in the morning can be a great way to wake you up and infuse your body with energy. The most notable breathing exercise right now is The Wim Hof Method. As a result of consistently exposing himself to extreme cold and heat, Wim Hof developed the method to withstand such conditions.

To begin to get comfortable, you can sit in a crossed-legged position or whatever you feel the most comfortable with. Just make sure that your lungs can expand without and restriction. For best results, practice when your stomach is empty.

Power - Close your eyes. Follow the same style of powerful short bursts of breathing as if you were blowing up a balloon. Inhale through the nose and exhale through the mouth. Maintain a consistent rhythm and allow your stomach to follow. Repeat for around thirty breaths. During this, you might feel light-headed, don't worry, it is normal.

Hold -After completing thirty rapid breaths, take in a deep breath to fill the lungs. Let the air out and then, in the end, hold it for as long as possible. Eventually, you will feel the gasp reflex. If you want to, you can add some push-ups while holding your breath. It will build your strength.

Recover - Bring the breath back in to fill your lungs and feel your chest expand. When you are filled with air, hold the breath for about ten seconds. It completes one round. Repeat for three rounds in succession.

The three steps process can be repeated in a cycle for around three rounds. After completion, take some time to relax and enjoy the feeling.

In addition to The Wim Hoff method or instead, you can try Tony Robbins' breathing technique. It infuses your body with energy. If you wake up feeling groggy and sluggish, try it out. Simple raise and lower your hands above your head as you breathe in and out explosively. Breathe in through the nose and out through the mouth. Repeat for thirty times and do three rounds. In between each round, jump lightly up and down and hum for ten to twenty times. Your body will wake up for sure.

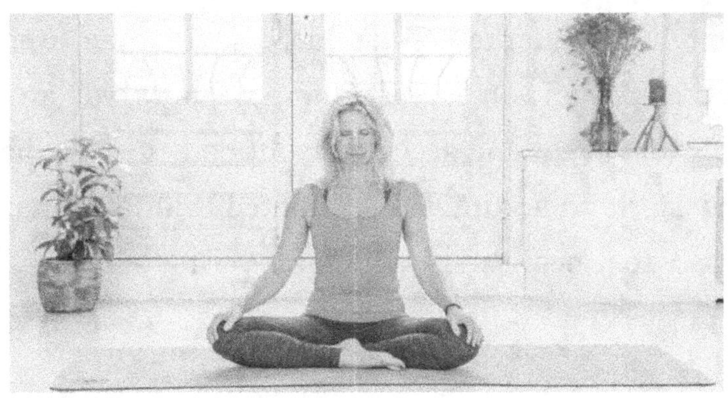

Chapter 16:
Overcome Emotional Food Cravings, How?

Candy, doughnuts, chocolate, pizza, pasta; there are tons of foods to choose from! We all get cravings for certain foods from time to time; the desire multiplies when you see your favorite food on the table. Food cravings are common amongst millions of people, and many find it extremely difficult to control, which ultimately leads to obesity and weight-gain issues. It is essential to understand that excessive eating causes disaster to your health in the long run.

The culprit for these cravings can be pinpointed to hormones. Hormones play a crucial role in every aspect of our life. They control our feelings, emotions, strengths, and weaknesses as well as our overall daily function. Hormones play a crucial role in increasing nighttime cravings. Once there feeding period has been completed, they immediately go to sleep right after consumption. It guarantees an increase in their weight for competition. When you eat just before sleeping, you are sure to increase your weight and accustom your body to "pre-diabetes." The body starts to accumulate unwanted calories, forcing your metabolism to process and burn them overnight.

Many people find it bewildering that even after a good dinner, the craving for more still exists. I was one of those people. I would consume a rather hearty dinner and always would be looking for more just hours later. The root cause is not an emotional imbalance or psychological disorder. It is pure biology. It all contributes to hormone, or rather problem in hormonal balance.

These hormones in your body change according to the different chemical reactions we undergo. Controlling them is crucial to ensure that they are working in a matter to benefit us rather than work against us. Any imbalance in their functionality leads to appetite instability. The most crucial hormones in overeating are Insulin, Leptin, Ghrelin,89765, and Peptide YY.

- **Insulin** – Insulin has a crucial role. It processes the sugar content from the food you eat. When there is a disturbance in its monitoring or functionality, it spikes and crashes. It will arise once you eat sugar or any junk food. An increase in insulin will make you hungry due to the release of insulin in your body.

- **Leptin** – Leptin functions as a hormone that communicates with the brain by telling it that the stomach is full. However, its functionality is prohibited with excessive intake of processed food. Over a period, the brain becomes leptin resistant, causing no action to the mind. The brain is unable to receive the signal that your stomach is full

- **Ghrelin** – This hormone is the appetite regulator. It monitors the body's requirement for food and sends the signal to the brain that the stomach is empty.

- **Peptide YY** – The Peptide hormone acts as a feedback to the stomach. The intestines produce the hormone, and they monitor your food intake. The hormone sends a signal of how full you are. It's only after your brain receives the message that you stop eating.

All these hormones work as sensors and help the brain regulate the functionality of your body, energy production, and hunger. When any one of these hormones are imbalanced, there is a misunderstanding, and the brain receives inappropriate information. During such instances, you will eat more even when you are full.

Overcoming cravings

Nighttime cravings are possible to overcome! You can get rid of them forever. It will, however, require you to be determined, consistent, and motivated to make this change. Here some keys step in reducing night time eating and binging.

1. **Breakfast:** Breakfast is an important meal of the day. It has a significant role in halting night time eating. Having a nutrient-filled breakfast will ensure your hormone levels are not altered. It will keep you going throughout the day and will set a tone for your body to follow. A common cause of nighttime binging is due to missing this critical meal to begin your day or not eating nutrient-filled foods.

To start with, ensure you have an adequate protein-rich breakfast. Try salads, fruits, juices, whole grain bread, and eggs. You can even get a protein shake. A fair shake is capable of balancing your sugar levels and keeping it even throughout the day.

2. **Liquids:** It is imperative to keep your body hydrated all the time. Water is a natural supplement for all humanity. You should have at least 1.2 liters (8 glasses) of water in a day. Try to keep away from drinks that are rich in calories such as sodas, lattes, iced teas, and coffee. Consuming these drinks spikes sugar levels and negatively effects the functioning of your hormones. Drinking such sugary liquids will make you crave food at night. Therefore, be very mindful of the fluids you consume.

3. **Eat less more often:** We often eat three meals a day. This long gap between meals initiates food cravings. Instead of having three big meals, concentrate on getting six meals. Reduce the consumption of the six meals. Eat less and increase the frequency. Such a process is highly efficient and helps the body get the essential nutrients at frequent intervals. You will also stay healthy and energetic all day.

4. **Eat last meal 3 hours before bedtime:** It is crucial to eat 2-3 hours before your bedtime. If you plan on staying up late and have gone more than 3 hours without food, you will binge. Cravings reach their peak when you start

going into "starvation mode." So, have a healthy snack late at night (Greek yogurt, protein shake, etc.); don't think of it as adding more calories, because this small meal will save you from eating a bag of chips.

5. **Stress**: Stress is your enemy. Keep away from it, or else you are bound to eat more. It would be best if you found your peace at all times. Find activities that will help you reduce your stress. Games, music, workout, and spending time with family are solutions through which you can conquer your stress. Learn different methods so that you can adapt to your workplace and stay at peace. Relaxing the mind, body, and soul is essential for overall health.

6. **Sleep pattern**: A good night's sleep is important for beginning the next day full of energy—improper sleep results in night cravings. When you do not have a proper sleep, the Ghrelin hormone reaches its peak, which results in the desire to eat late at night. The only method you can control it is by having a peaceful sleep. Sleeping earlier will help you get a night of restful sleep and lower your caloric intake. You can't eat at night if you're asleep!

7. **Supplements**: Supplements are natural molecules that help balance your hormones. The following are good for overall health:

   a) **Omega-3 Fats:** Fish and fish oil are rich in Omega-3 fats. You can eat them in the form of food or capsules. One capsule a day is enough to keep the momentum and balance.

b) **Vitamin D**: Vitamin D helps in balancing insulin. It also monitors and regulates the functioning of your hormones.

c) **PGX**: PGX is a fiber supplement. Seaweed and Glucomannan are great supplements to use. This supplement is available as a powder and in capsules. It has an excellent effect on cutting your night cravings. Consume a capsule 15 minutes before dinner. Take another pill after completing your dinner. It reduces the spike of insulin, which results in the slow functioning of the hormone. It will result in achieving a full stomach. The high fiber supplement creates a balance of your hormones, which assists in reducing night cravings. You are

8. **Gum:** When a night time craving hits, chew some gum. I know it sounds simple enough, but many times we are just looking for a taste of something sweet. We are not hungry but want to keep our mouth busy. Chewing gum will satisfy your appetite and is an easy solution.

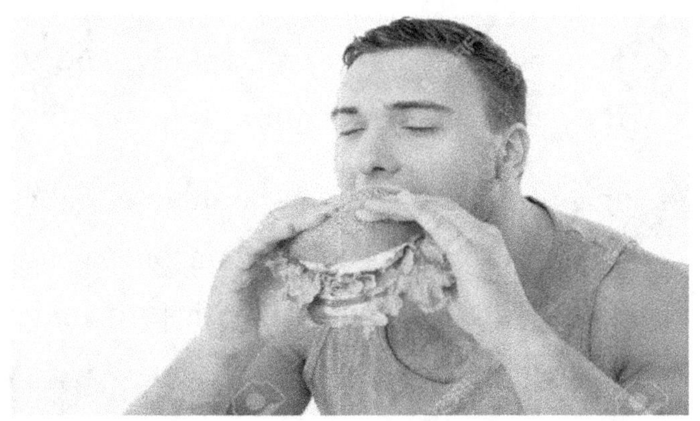

Chapter 17:
Become organic

It's NOT a good idea to decide out of desperation. There are many weight loss techniques hidden in plain sight that are scientifically-backed, natural, and inexpensive.

Because weight loss is a big market, it's common to get sold things like diet pills of dubious origin, expensive surgeries, or weight loss regiments that are "proven to work" with alluring before and after photos. Or how about those pills that say "No lifestyle change required! Just take the pill and watch the weight disappear!"

Medically speaking, this is, of course, impossible unless the pill in question is a tapeworm. And I promise you don't want to be taking that (even though it is a "natural cure," I suppose).

So what do these practices tell you about the weight loss industry?

It indicates that you need to tread carefully, and when on a diet—stick to the basics and seek natural solutions first.

I do believe some of the latest understandings about weight loss are "revolutionary." From hacking your body's metabolism, creating constant calorie-burning activities, to understanding emotional and mental links to weight gain. Today we better understand why it's easier for some people to shed pounds versus others, and these new techniques and so-called "hacks" could make burning calories much easier for new generations.

Besides, because of the expanding field of epigenetics, we are learning how we are not entirely slaves to our genetic code. The idea that some of us are "genetically cursed" to get fat/stay fat is not true. It has significant consequences in many areas of medicine, including weight loss.

I think the reason so many look for "natural solutions" to weight loss, and why it's ultimately the best way to create real solutions, is because we have to work within the parameters of nature to be able to heal any aspect of ourselves. The alternative is to get burned by Big Pharma and the mainstream medical world that cruelly / mercilessly exploits people. While weight loss surgery, diet pills, and other techniques may even yield some results—at what cost to your body and your long-term health?

The world of ANY natural alternative or supplement that exists outside of the spectrum of FDA approval is going to be fraught with charlatans. You need to keep a critical mind and also stay scientifically minded.

For instance, you may hear some natural salesmen come out with the latest "big idea" that a previously thought uninteresting ingredient now magically transforms overweight people into runway models.

Because there's a demand for new fads, people will meet that demand by stretching the truth. The only way to tell what's real and what isn't is to drill down and get the facts behind certain products.

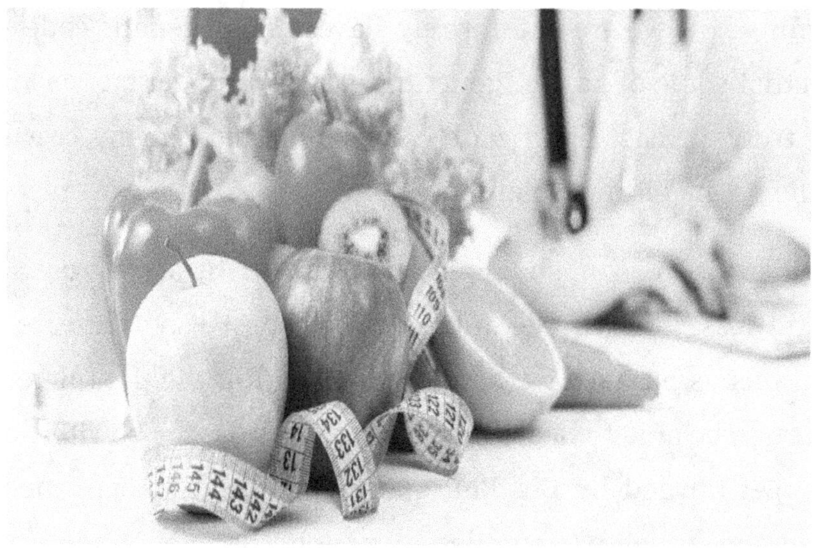

Chapter 18:
Simple Substitutions for Healthier Food

Replace Sugar with Honey

Honey is one of the natural sweeteners that have been approved worldwide as a substitute for sugar. Honey is recommended for two main reasons; it is twice as sweet as sugar and tons of times possesses more nutritional value. Though honey contains as many calories as sugar, it contains, however, simple sugars that can easily be absorbed into the blood system; these include fructose. Honey has a broader application as compared to sugar; sugar, for instance, has no medicinal value.

Honey has anti-microbial activities, and that is why it is used in MRSA in hospitals. From researches, it can be confirmed that 100g of sugar contains much more calories than 100g of honey; this honey can help you manage your weight much easier while sugar contributes to weight gain significantly. Honey includes more than 15% of water, which is more than water found in sugar, and this also accounts for its less calorie value (granulated sugar has no water). A hundred grams of granulated sugar can provide 1620kj, while the same amount of honey provides 1273kj of energy.

Granulated sugar can be described as 100% carbohydrate, but sugars found in honey are different. While most carbs found in sugar are sucrose and the rest glucose and fructose, honey, on the other hand, only contains 1.5g of sucrose, and the rest are fructose and glucose within a 100g of honey. When an athlete needs brief and sustained energy, he or she will instead opt for honey than sugar because of the composition of easy, simple sugars in honey.

One of the benefits of substituting sugar with honey when dieting is that honey can help sustain your energy levels. However, you must not consume too much of honey. While sugar contains no essential vitamins, honey comes with some; for instance, a 100g of honey contains about 1% of vitamin C and 1% of niacin. Honey is also believed to contain excellent quality proteins. 100g of honey, for instance, provides 0.3g of protein, which makes it much better than sugar that contains none. Though honey has the recommended mineral elements such as; calcium, iron, magnesium, phosphorous, zinc, sodium, and manganese, such mineral elements are not sufficient enough for your daily dose. Honey has 4% manganese and 2% iron, whereas sugar only provides 1% selenium.

Honey is beneficial for weight loss because it provides you sustainable energy; however, honey should be substituted only in place of sugar because it still has a high amount of calories, though it is more nutritious.

There is no doubt to the fact that honey has a much better sweetening effect than sugar; for instance, you may need a tablespoon of honey in place of three teaspoons of sugar for the same purpose. Sugar has more calories than honey; thus, the more you add, the more sharply your calorie intake increases while honey helps you maintain a stable calorie level. The more you dilute honey, the more its sweetness diminishes; however, its main vitamins, and minerals as well as antibiotic activities, will remain. It, however, does not mean you must be reckless with honey. Experts recommend that you should not take more than two teaspoons of honey at a time, because it can affect your teeth when taken excessively for a very long time.

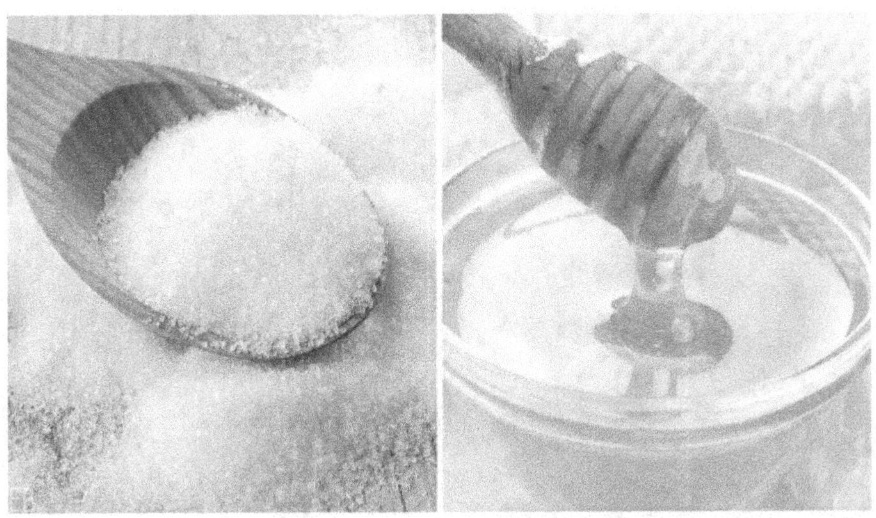

Chapter 19:
Turn on the lights

People who eat in well-lit spaces **consume about 39 percent fewer calories**-and make healthier food choices than those who dine under dim lighting, says recent research. Why? Bright areas make us feel more alert, so we nosh more mindfully. Participants who skipped the candles at mealtime ate more slowly, enjoyed their food more, and, yes, ate 373 fewer calories.

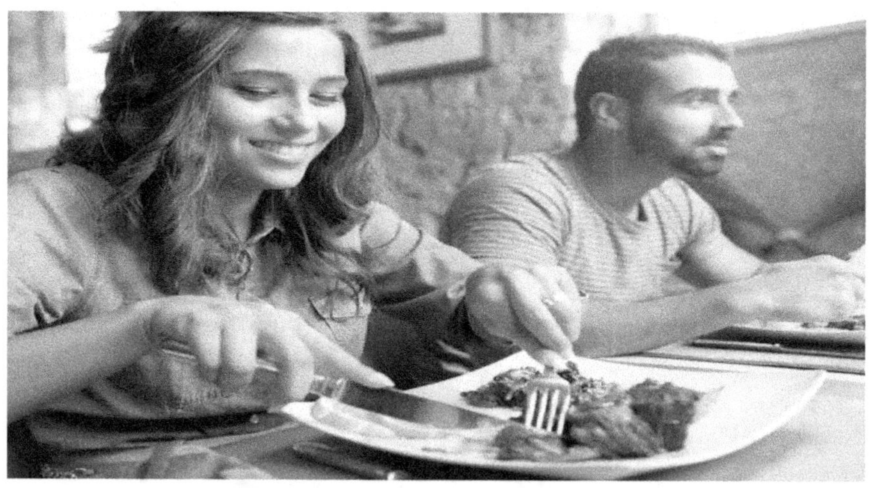

Chapter 20:
Snack on Yogurt

Yogurt was recently identified as a top weight-loss-promoting food by Harvard University. It's high in protein, which, gram for gram, helps fill you up more than carbs. Stick to plain yogurt for a healthy snack, without lots of added sugar, and add fresh fruit to sweeten your cup. Another bonus? The probiotics in yogurt may help you burn fat. In one study, researchers gave overweight but otherwise healthy adults about 1/2 cup of yogurt at dinner every night for six weeks. Some ate yogurt supplemented with an added dose of probiotics (either Lactobacillus fermentum or L. amylovorus), while others got regular yogurt (which has a lower probiotic content). Though none of the subjects lost weight, those consuming the probiotic-enriched yogurt lost 3 to 4 percent of their body fat, compared to just 1 percent body fat lost in the other group. To ensure your yogurt delivers a decent amount of probiotics, look for one that carries the "Live & Active Cultures" seal.

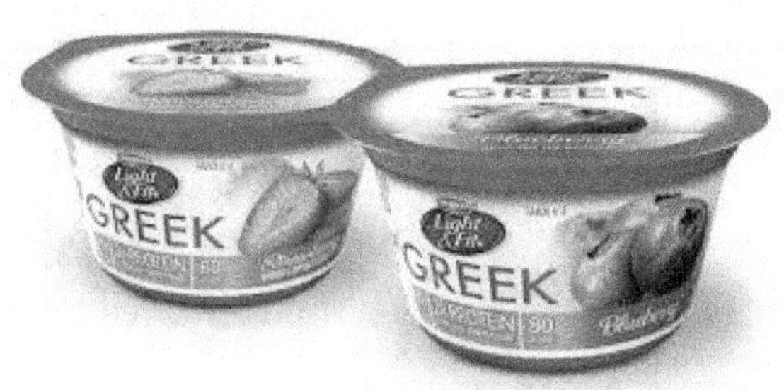

Chapter 21:
Reduce inflammation by eating this food

Gaining weight, or the inability to shed excess pounds, is often a red flag that there is underlying low-grade inflammation in the body. And on the flip side, even the most **disciplined eating and exercise habits are often ineffective** when inflammation is present. At the same time, the dynamic between weight and inflammation is complicated, research points toward reducing inflammation as being as integral to weight loss as diet and activity. So what are the best double-duty foods, the ones that reduce inflammation while also supporting weight loss? Here the 10 top anti-inflammatory foods for weight loss.

Cauliflower or broccoli "rice": Swapping out carb-rich foods like pasta and rice for riced cauliflower or broccoli can help cut calories and carbs and to help soothe inflammation. When finely chopped, these two low-carb veggies provide a grain-like base for creamy or saucy dishes or can be sautéed with other veggies to great a low-carb stir-fry. And because cauliflower and broccoli are part of the cruciferous vegetable family, they contain various plant compounds that may have powerful anti-inflammatory effects when eaten regularly.

Berries: Contains fiber. This fiber helps provide a feeling of fullness, and it also means berries tend to have a lower glycemic response compared to many other fruits, which is good for blood sugar management, cravings, and inflammation. Another perk is their hefty dose of antioxidants and anthocyanins, which help tamp down existing and future inflammation.

Walnuts: Eating a combination of fiber, protein, and healthy fat at meals and snacks is a game-changer when dieting because of the satiety this combo provides. And tree nuts like walnuts, almonds, and pistachios have an ideal balance of all three nutrients, including some anti-inflammatory omega-3 fats.

Greek yogurt: Choose Greek yogurt for higher levels of protein (and opt for plain instead of flavored to avoid added sugars). Then add fresh fruit or nuts for a little sweetness and crunch.

Beans: High-fiber beans and legumes like black beans, navy beans, chickpeas, peas, and lentils are good sources of both protein and slow-digesting carbohydrates. This combination offers short-term benefits by leaving the stomach full and preventing sudden glucose spikes, and also appears to have long-term weight loss benefits.

Leafy greens: Aim to get in the habit of adding a handful or two of leafy greens like baby spinach, kale, arugula, lettuces, and other greens to your plate at most meals, whether it's in the form of a salad or mixed in with other ingredients.

Avocado: Not only is this creamy fruit full of monounsaturated fats, vitamin E, fiber, and carotenoids, which collectively work together to soothe inflammation in the body, but research suggests that people who eat avocado daily tend to have lower body weights and lower BMIs. These statistically significant results were in comparison to those who rarely ate avocado or had much less frequent consumption.

Extra-virgin olive oil: All fats and oils have approximately the same calories and fat per tablespoon, but olive oil is a good source of those healthier unsaturated fats and contains a unique compound called oleocanthal , which has anti-inflammatory effects in the body. All olive oils contain oleocanthal, but less-refined types like extra-virgin have higher levels, so make that you are go-to for salad dressings and when cooking at lower heats.

Garlic and spices: By incorporating garlic and spices like turmeric, rosemary, cinnamon, cumin, and ginger, you'll prevent meal fatigue, as well as calm inflammation. While fragrant spices and pungent garlic may seem like they have the potential to aggravate inflammation, research suggests they do the opposite. Their aromatic compounds have been used medically in other cultures for years for anti-inflammatory effects.

Citrus fruit: Choosing fiber-rich foods like citrus may also offer some additional weight-loss perks when it comes to sleep. Research suggests that eating a low-fiber diet is associated with decreased sleep quality. It is important because inadequate sleep triggers changes that can reduce insulin sensitivity and increase appetite and risk of weight gain. So getting a serving of citrus each day is a low-calorie way to get more fiber, as well as load up on vitamin C, which is an antioxidant that prevents inflammation.

Chapter 22:
Try different cooking methods, such as grilling, roasting, baking, or poaching.

Preparing your meals at home is recommended as you can regulate the amount of oil or fats you use. This aids in weight loss. Some of the best cooking methods that reduce fat include:

Steaming- When steaming food, you do not need to add fats or oil that may eventually cause weight gain. It is a suitable method of cooking as it seals in the moisture and flavour of food while cooking while preserving its nutritional value.

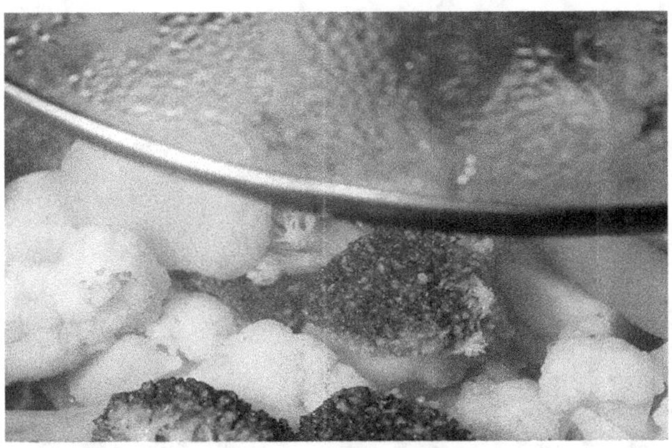

Poaching - In this method, food is cooked by submerging it in liquid. The liquid can be water, milk, wine or Stock. This cooking technique is ideal for delicate foods like eggs, poultry, fish, or fruit as it uses a relatively low temperature compared to other "moist heat" cooking methods. Poaching does not use fat or oil for cooking; hence considered a healthy cooking technique.

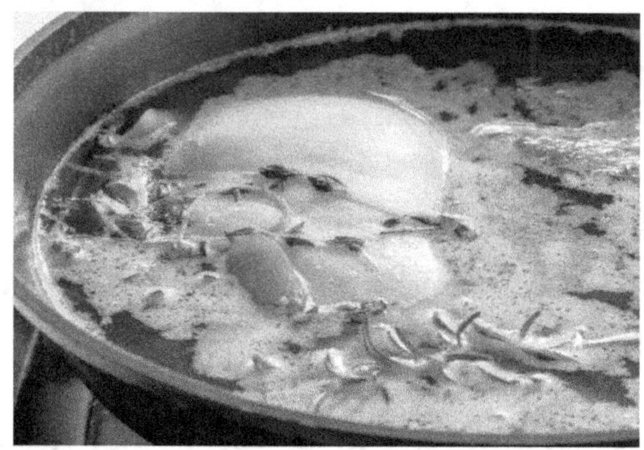

Grilling- This technique is usually used for cooking meat and vegetables. It uses direct heat applied to the surface of the food either from above, below, or on the sided. The heat source could be charcoal fire, ceramic briquettes heated by gas flames. No oil is used when grilling.

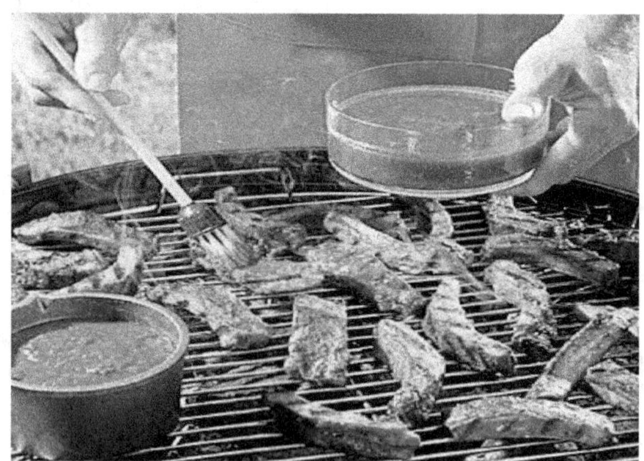

Conclusion

Losing weight can be one of the most tedious tasks for an individual if he or she does not use the appropriate measures and techniques. Usually, individuals look towards diet control programs that constitute complicated meal plans that promise to make the user lose weight in a relatively shorter amount of time. The other popular mode of weight loss most individuals resorts to are vigorous physical exercise routines that often push the users beyond their limits to help achieve their ideal weight. In either case, these weight loss regimes can be exhausting and tend to drain the person halfway through and even manage to irritate the users due to their complex and rigid steps.

What must be realized is that weight loss is a steady process that should involve the user changing his or her lifestyle gradually in such a manner that they can sustain those habits. The methods applied for losing all the extra weight should be unproblematic and straightforward for the users. Keeping all that in mind we bring to you this eBook that is divided into four chapters containing a total of twenty easy to do steps that will not only help shed those extra pounds but will also help bring a healthy more positive approach towards life